I0467893

Autoimmune Cookbook

Autoimmune All-Day Recipes Vol. 2

All Rights Reserved. No part of this publication may be reproduced in any form or by any means, including scanning, photocopying, or otherwise without prior written permission of the copyright holder. Copyright © 2014

About the Author – Melissa Groves

Melissa graduated from Hofstra University with a BA in English and Dance. As a dancer, she was always interested in nutrition and how to make healthy foods taste good. For over 15 years, he had a successful career in NYC as an advertising copywriter, but decided to leave that world to pursue her true passion, nutrition. She currently lives in New Hampshire, where she is going back to school, with the goal of becoming a registered dietitian. She is a 2000 graduate of the Institute for Integrative Nutrition. Her recipes have won national awards.

Table of Contents

Why the Autoimmune Protocol?

Every day, dozens of people across the country get diagnosed with one or more autoimmune condition: systemic lupus erythematosus, celiac disease, Graves' disease, rheumatoid arthritis, type 1 diabetes… All these conditions and many more are caused by a dysfunction of the immune system. Normally, the immune system is responsible for fighting off microorganisms such as viruses, bacteria and fungi that would otherwise invade our bodies. However, some people's immune system has difficulty differentiating between self and non-self. Essentially, these people's immune system attacks their own body tissues. Some auto-immune diseases destroy the intestines, while others destroy joints, organs, skin or glands.

Science doesn't know the exact reasons why some people's immune system will attack healthy body tissues. What we do know is that many autoimmune reactions are in fact a response to a trigger: drugs, viruses or bacteria, irritants, food, etc. For example, someone with celiac disease will suffer intestinal damage after eating food that contains gluten (a protein found in wheat, barley and rye). Other people are sensitive to specific vegetables, chemicals or environmental triggers that cause heavy inflammation in their joints. In other words, autoimmune conditions seem to be similar to allergies, but with chronic consequences rather than an immediate reactions such as those seen when people come in contact with allergens. This leads the scientific community to further try to understand the role of inflammation in autoimmunity.

There are strong beliefs that some specific foods are more likely to trigger autoimmune reactions. These foods contain certain toxins, proteins or molecules that cause inflammation and trigger autoimmune reactions. This interesting topic has led to the creation of a very restrictive diet designed to eliminate all the common inflammation-causing "problem foods" from one's diet and reintroduce them one at a time in order to identify the culprit(s). This diet is known as the autoimmune protocol (AIP). The goal of the autoimmune protocol is to allow the person's immune system to rest, lower inflammation levels and allow for recovery. Once inflammation levels are low enough and the gut is healed, the person can start reintroducing foods one by one, carefully monitoring any resulting autoimmune flare-ups. Since the autoimmune protocol is generally pretty boring, most people are excited to reintroduce foods after several weeks.

It is important to *avoid cheating* while on the AIP. A small slip-up could ruin your efforts at trying to figure out which foods are causing your immune system to attack your own body. Healing from the damage done by inflammation is extremely important: chronic inflammation can lead to pain, loss of mobility, organ failure and several other potentially serious complications. Inflammation is the result of the immune system's attempt at eradicating a "threat" (the food you're eating) by launching a generalized inflammation attack all over your tissues and organs. Most people feel significantly better on the AIP and many decide to keep an anti-inflammatory diet for the rest of their lives. The Paleolithic diet is a very popular follow-up to the autoimmune protocol because of its major health benefits on inflammation levels.

How should you reintroduce foods? The key is to start small. Have a bite, then have a large portion of it later the same day. You need to eat enough of it to create a response. If you haven't responded after 4-5 days, chances are that you have no antibodies against that specific food. It can be considered safe and added to your regular diet. If you react to a food, it needs to be banned as it will nearly always trigger your immune system, much like an allergic person will always react to peanuts/shrimp/pollen/etc. Reactions can widely vary in nature, from "brain fog" and lethargy to insomnia, depression and disease flare-ups.

The autoimmune protocol is a very basic diet. It consists of fruits, vegetables and meat. However, not all vegetables are allowed: a specific family of vegetables known as nightshades causes autoimmune reactions in a large amount of people. The nightshade family includes eggplants, tomatoes, peppers (sweet and hot kinds – even chilies and jalapeños), mustard and potatoes. Artificial and no-calorie sweeteners are banned, as are processed foods, vegetable oils, dairy, grains, nuts, seeds, legumes, eggs, dried fruit and alcohol. What you can eat: meat (preferably grass-fed), fish and seafood, around 2 pieces of fruit per day, the occasional use of natural sweeteners (maple syrup, honey) in small amounts, fermented foods, many coconut products including milk, oil and coconut aminos, clarified butter (known as ghee) and non-nightshade veggies. Fats such as olive oil, lard and bacon fat are allowed, as are avocadoes, herbs, green tea and vinegar.

Since sticking to the autoimmune protocol is the key to its success, it is important to gather as much information as possible before starting. Of course, a cookbook containing creative autoimmune-friendly recipes is also a handy addition to your kitchen, as you will soon realize that you can't cook most of your favorite meals. Having such a cookbook can make following AIP guidelines easier as well. You can make AIP meals enjoyable by thinking outside the box and this cookbook is here to accomplish just that: inspire you to create healthy, anti-inflammatory meals that will make you feel truly great.

Foods to Avoid

You will want to avoid:

- Anything pre-packaged, canned or boxed, including frozen entrees and prepared salads or sandwiches. Most pre-packaged foods contain foods to avoid and are heavily processed. Canned or frozen veggies (excluding tomatoes) and pre-packaged baby spinach or lettuce mixes are generally fine
- No-calorie sweeteners and sugar substitutes, including stevia, xylitol and other sugar alcohols, sucralose, aspartame, acesulfame-k
- Added sugar (soda, candy and chocolate are obvious, but sugar is in everything including vinaigrettes and canned vegetables)
- All grains: wheat, barley, rye, rice, quinoa, amaranth, buckwheat, wild rice, oats, kamut, millet, sorghum, etc.
- Dairy, including butter, cheese, milk and yogurt. The *only* exception is cultured ghee (clarified butter, certified free of casein and lactose)
- Alcohol and excess caffeine (green tea is fine)
- Eggs
- Legumes: all dried beans, chickpeas, soy, edamame, hummus, etc. Green and string beans are fine
- Nuts and their oils
- Seeds and their oils: chia, flax, hemp, seed-based spices such as cumin and coriander, mustard, nutmeg, caraway, poppyseed

- Dried fruit and fructose (2 pieces of fresh fruit per day are acceptable)
- Nightshades: potatoes, tomatoes, sweet peppers (green, yellow, red, orange), hot peppers, chilies, eggplant
- Vegetable oils, except olive and coconut

Chapter 1

Soups and Salads

Creamy Parsnip Soup

Prep Time: 10 minutes

Cook Time: 25 minutes

Servings: 4

INGREDIENTS

1 large yellow onion, chopped

2 ripe pears, peeled and chopped

6 parsnips, peeled and chopped

4 cups chicken or vegetable broth

2 Tablespoons olive oil

1 teaspoon sea salt

INSTRUCTIONS

1. Sauté onion in olive oil in a large stockpot over medium-high heat until translucent.
2. Add parsnips, pears, broth, and salt.
3. Cover and bring to a boil.
4. Reduce heat to medium and simmer for approximately 20 minutes, until parsnips are tender.
5. Puree the soup with a hand blender, or in batches in a blender or food processor.

Chicken Soup

Prep Time: 10 minutes

Cook Time: 40 minutes

Servings: 4

INGREDIENTS

1 large yellow onion, chopped

4 garlic cloves, minced

2 carrots, chopped

2 stalks of celery, chopped

1 cup sliced mushrooms

½ cup parsley, chopped

4 cups chicken broth

2 skinless chicken legs

2 skinless chicken thighs

2 Tablespoons olive oil

1 teaspoon sea salt

INSTRUCTIONS

1. Sauté onion and garlic in olive oil in a large stockpot over medium heat until translucent.
2. Add the celery, carrots, and mushrooms and cook, stirring, for about 5 minutes.
3. Add the chicken legs and thighs, broth, parsley, and salt. Cover and simmer for 30 minutes.

4. Remove the chicken from the pot and pull the meat off the bones. Chop the meat and add it back to the pot. Simmer another 5 minutes, then serve.

Emerald Soup

Prep Time: 10 minutes

Cook Time: 25 minutes

Servings: 4

INGREDIENTS

2 large leeks, sliced

2 Tablespoons fresh ginger, grated

4 garlic cloves, minced

2 cups Chinese cabbage, chopped

4 cups fresh spinach

4 cups chicken or vegetable broth

2 Tablespoons coconut oil

1 teaspoon sea salt

INSTRUCTIONS

1. Sauté leeks in coconut oil in a large stockpot over medium-high heat about 5 minutes.
2. Add ginger and garlic, and stir, cooking, for another minute.
3. Add the cabbage, broth, and salt. Cover, and simmer for 20 minutes.
4. Add the spinach and stir in until wilted.

Citrus Fennel Salad

Prep Time: minutes

Chill time: 20 minutes

Servings: 4

INGREDIENTS

4 cups radicchio, chopped

2 fennel bulbs

4 oranges, peeled and sectioned

1 lemon, juiced (about 2 Tablespoons)

2 Tablespoons olive oil

Sea salt to taste

INSTRUCTIONS

1. Trim the fennel, removing the leaves and roots. Slice each bulb into thin slices, then cut into bite-sized pieces and place into a bowl.
2. Cut the oranges into bite-sized pieces and add them to the bowl.
3. Add the lemon juice, olive oil, and salt to the bowl and toss to combine. Chill for at least 20 minutes.
4. Serve the salad on top of the radicchio.

Pineapple Jicama Salad

Prep Time: minutes

Cook Time: N/A

Servings: 4

INGREDIENTS

1 small red onion, thinly sliced

2 cups jicama, peeled and diced

2 cups pineapple, peeled, cored, and chopped

4 cups red cabbage, shredded

2 Tablespoons lime juice

2 Tablespoons olive oil

½ cup fresh mint leaves

1 teaspoon sea salt

INSTRUCTIONS

1. In a bowl, combine the onion, jicama, pineapple, and mint.
2. In a separate bowl, whisk the olive oil, lime juice, and salt.
3. Serve the salad on a bed of red cabbage and drizzle the dressing over it before serving.

Chapter 2

Main Dishes

Steak Tacos

Prep Time: 10 minutes

Cook Time: 10 minutes

Servings: 4

INGREDIENTS

8 large lettuce leaves

3 Tablespoons olive oil

1 pound skirt steak or flank steak

½ bunch cilantro, chopped

8 radishes, chopped

4 scallions, chopped

1 teaspoon sea salt

INSTRUCTIONS

1. Heat 1 Tablespoon of oil in a large skillet over high. Cook the steak for 5 minutes on each side.
2. Wash the lettuce and pat the leaves dry with paper towels.
3. In a bowl, combine the radishes, scallions, cilantro, lime juice, and 2 Tablespoons of olive oil.
4. Fill each of the lettuce leaves with the steak and top with the radish mixture.

Steak with Mushroom Sauce

Prep Time: 10 minutes

Cook Time: 25 minutes

Servings: 2

INGREDIENTS

4 Tablespoons olive oil

2 NY strip steaks (8-10 ounces each)

4 ounces cremini mushrooms, sliced

4 ounces Portobello mushrooms, sliced

4 ounces shiitake mushrooms, sliced

1 shallot, thinly sliced

1 teaspoon tarragon

¼ cup AIP-friendly balsamic vinegar

1 cup beef broth

1 teaspoon sea salt

INSTRUCTIONS

1. Heat 2 Tablespoon of oil in a large skillet over high.
2. Season the steaks with salt and sear for 4 minutes on each side over medium heat.
3. Remove the steaks from the pan, and cover.
4. In the same pan, sauté the shallot in 2 tablespoons oil until translucent.
5. Add the mushrooms and tarragon and sauté until the mushrooms begin to soften, about 5 minutes.

6. Add the balsamic vinegar and broth. Cook until the liquid is reduced by half, about 8-10 minutes.

7. Serve the steaks topped with the mushroom sauce.

Skillet Sausage Scramble

Prep Time: 10 minutes

Cook Time: 35 minutes

Servings: 4

INGREDIENTS

2 Tablespoons coconut oil

1 small yellow onion, diced

16 ounces sausage, chopped

1 large sweet potato, peeled and diced

2 cups baby spinach

¼ cup water

Sea salt to taste

½ teaspoon cinnamon (optional)

INSTRUCTIONS

1. Sauté the onion in the oil in a large skillet over medium-high heat until just starting to brown, about 5 minutes.
2. Add the sausage and sauté until browned, about 10 minutes.
3. Add the sweet potato, water, and cinnamon (if using). Cover and cook until the sweet potato is tender, 10-15 minutes.
4. Remove cover and stir in spinach. Stir until spinach is wilted.

"Spaghetti" and Meatballs

Prep Time: 20 minutes

Cook Time: 30 minutes

Servings: 4

INGREDIENTS

1 large spaghetti squash

2 pounds ground beef

4 cloves garlic, minced

2 teaspoons olive oil

½ cup fresh parsley, chopped

½ teaspoon sea salt

INSTRUCTIONS

1. Preheat oven to 400 °F.
2. Cut spaghetti squash in half lengthwise, scoop out the seeds, and place cut-side down on a baking sheet lightly coated with 1 teaspoon of olive oil. Pierce the skin several times with a fork.
3. Put the spaghetti squash in the oven and bake for 15 minutes.
4. While the squash bakes, combine the beef, garlic, parsley, and ½ teaspoon salt in a large bowl with your hands. Roll into meatballs, approximately 1-1/2 inches in diameter.
5. Place the meatballs on a baking sheet lightly coated with 1 teaspoon of olive oil.
6. Add the meatballs to the oven and bake alongside the squash for 15 minutes.

7. When the spaghetti squash is done and cool enough to handle, scrape out the strands with a fork into a large bowl (you may want to hold the squash using an oven mitt while you do this).
8. Serve the spaghetti squash with the meatballs and Italian Red Sauce (recipe below).

Italian Red Sauce

Prep Time: 10 minutes

Cook Time: 1 hour and 20 minutes

Servings: Makes about 4 cups

INGREDIENTS

3 cups vegetable stock

1 medium butternut squash, peeled, seeded, and cut into chunks

2 beets, peeled and chopped

1 large onion, chopped

4 cloves garlic, minced

2 Tablespoons apple cider vinegar

1 bay leaf

1 teaspoon dried basil

1 teaspoon dried oregano

1 teaspoon dried parsley

½ teaspoon dried thyme

3 Tablespoons olive oil

INSTRUCTIONS

1. Sauté the onion in the oil in a large stockpot over medium-high heat until just starting to brown, about 5 minutes.

2. Add the squash, beets, garlic, and 2 cups of the broth. Cook until the vegetables are tender, about 30 minutes.

3. Puree the mixture with a hand blender, or in batches in a blender or food processor.

4. Add the pureed mixture back to the stockpot. Add the spices, the rest of the broth, and the vinegar and simmer over low heat until thickened, about another 30-45 minutes.

5. Serve over any autoimmune-friendly pasta substitute.

Mahi Mahi with Citrus Salsa

Prep Time: 10 minutes

Cook Time: 10 minutes

Servings: 2

INGREDIENTS

1 pound fresh mahi mahi fillets

1 Tablespoon coconut oil

1 grapefruit

2 oranges

1 lemon

1 lime

1 tablespoon minced red onion

¼ cup chopped fresh cilantro

½ teaspoon sea salt

INSTRUCTIONS

1. Sear the fish in the oil in a skillet over medium high heat, 3-4 minutes per side, until golden brown. Let rest 5-10 minutes.
2. With a sharp knife, remove the skin and the white pith from all of the fruit. Cut between the membranes and transfer the fruit to a bowl, removing any seeds.
3. Toss the fruit with the onion, cilantro, and salt.
4. Serve the salsa over the fish.

Cod with Saffron and Garlic

Prep Time: 5 minutes

Cook Time: 15 minutes

Servings: 2

INGREDIENTS

1 pound fresh cod fillets

2 Tablespoons olive oil

4 garlic cloves, thinly sliced

1 shallot, thinly sliced

Pinch of saffron threads

1 Tablespoon lemon juice

½ teaspoon dried parsley

Lemon wedges for serving (optional)

1 teaspoon sea salt

INSTRUCTIONS

1. In a skillet, sauté the garlic and shallots in oil until translucent.
2. Add the fish to the skillet.
3. Mix the saffron, lemon juice, parsley, and salt in a small bowl and pour over the fish.
4. Cover the skillet and cook on low heat for about 10 minutes, until fish is opaque and flakes easily.
5. Serve with lemon wedges.

Quick Chicken Stir-Fry

Prep Time: 15 minutes

Cook Time: 20 minutes

Servings: 4

INGREDIENTS

1 pound chicken meat, cut into 1-inch chunks

1 yellow onion, sliced

2 carrots, peeled and sliced thinly

4 cups baby bok choy (about 2 heads), chopped

12 ounces mushrooms, halved

4 Tablespoons coconut oil

4 cloves garlic, chopped

1 Tablespoon grated ginger

1 Tablespoon apple cider vinegar.

1 teaspoon sea salt

INSTRUCTIONS

1. Sauté onions in coconut oil in a deep sauté pan or wok for about 3 minutes, or until translucent.
2. Add the chicken and cook, stirring frequently, until lightly browned.
3. Add the bok choy, carrots, and mushrooms and continue to sauté for a few minutes.
4. In a separate bowl, mix the vinegar, garlic, ginger, and salt, and whisk until blended.

5. Pour the sauce over the chicken and vegetables and cook, stirring frequently until vegetables are crisp-tender.

Pork Tenderloin with Apples

Prep Time: 10 minutes

Cook Time: 40 minutes

Servings: 4

INGREDIENTS

2 pork tenderloins (3/4 to 1 pound)

¼ cup apple cider vinegar

4 red apples, peeled and sliced

2 Tablespoons coconut oil

1 cup chicken or beef broth

1 teaspoon sea salt

½ teaspoon cinnamon (optional)

INSTRUCTIONS

1. Preheat oven to 400 °F.
2. Heat the oil in a skillet on medium high. Add the tenderloins and sear on all sides (about 10 minutes). Do not discard the juices in the skillet.
3. Place the tenderloins in a roasting pan, add the broth and vinegar, and place in the oven for 10 minutes.
4. Cook the apples in the same skillet used for the pork. Add the cinnamon, if using, and cook until soft.
5. Remove the apples from the pan, again reserving the juices in the skillet.
6. Remove the roast from the oven, transfer the tenderloins to a cutting board, and pour the roasting juices into the skillet.

7. Heat all of the liquid in the skillet over high heat, until the consistency of gravy (about 10 minutes).

8. Slice the tenderloin into thin pieces and serve with the apple slices. Drizzle the gravy over all.

Turkey Cutlets

Prep Time: 5 minutes

Cook Time: 20 minutes

Servings: 4

INGREDIENTS

2 pounds sliced raw turkey cutlets

4 Tablespoons olive oil

2 garlic cloves, sliced

1 cup chicken broth

1 Tablespoon lemon juice

2 Tablespoons capers

¼ cup fresh parsley, chopped.

½ teaspoon sea salt

INSTRUCTIONS

1. Heat turkey in 3 Tablespoons oil in a heavy skillet over high heat. Cook the turkey until brown on both sides and cooked through, about 3 minutes per side. Transfer turkey to a plate, and cover to keep warm.

2. Add remaining oil to the skillet and sauté the garlic. Add the broth and cook over medium-high heat, until reduced to about ¾ cup. Stir in lemon juice, capers, parsley, and sea salt.

3. Return the turkey to the skillet and cook until heated through, about 1-2 minutes.

Chapter 3

Side Dishes

Lemon-Vinaigrette Carrots

Prep Time: 5 minutes

Cook Time: 5 minutes

Servings: 4

INGREDIENTS

1 pound baby carrots

½ cup olive oil

¼ cup lemon juice

1 garlic clove, minced

½ teaspoon dried parsley

½ teaspoon sea salt

INSTRUCTIONS

1. Steam carrots in a steamer insert or in about ½-inch of water until tender, 5-7 minutes.
2. Whisk the oil, lemon juice, and remaining ingredients in a small bowl.
3. Drain the carrots and toss with the dressing.

Sautéed Southern-Style Greens

Prep Time: 10 minutes

Cook Time: 15 minutes

Servings: 4

INGREDIENTS

2 bunches collard greens, sliced into thin ribbons

3 Tablespoons olive oil or bacon fat

1 yellow onion, thinly sliced

4 cloves garlic, thinly sliced

1 Tablespoon apple cider vinegar

1 teaspoon sea salt

4 strips cooked bacon (optional)

INSTRUCTIONS

1. Sauté onions in oil or fat in a large skillet over medium-high heat until translucent. Add the garlic and cook for another minute, stirring frequently.
2. Add the greens and cover. Cook until the greens are wilted, about 5-7 minutes.
3. Remove the cover, add the vinegar and salt, and continue to cook, stirring frequently until greens are cooked down and soft.
4. Crumble the bacon over the greens (if using) and serve.

Mashed Root Vegetables

Prep Time: 15 minutes

Cook Time: 30 minutes

Servings: 4

INGREDIENTS

2 parsnips

1 medium celery root

2 turnips

1 sweet potato

2 Tablespoons olive oil

2 tablespoons chicken broth

Sea salt to taste

INSTRUCTIONS

1. Peel and chop all of the vegetables.
2. In a medium, saucepan, bring the vegetables to a boil in about 2 quarts of water. Cover and cook until tender, about 20 minutes.
3. Drain the vegetables and return them to the pot. Add the olive oil and chicken broth and mash, using a potato masher. Add salt to taste.

Stuffed Acorn Squash

Prep Time: 15 minutes

Cook Time: 45 minutes

Servings: 4

INGREDIENTS

2 large acorn squash

2 carrots, chopped

2 turnips, chopped

2 apples, peeled and chopped

½ teaspoon ground cinnamon

2 Tablespoons coconut oil

1 teaspoon sea salt

1 teaspoon olive oil

INSTRUCTIONS

1. Preheat oven to 400 °F.
2. Cut the squash in half, from top to bottom. Scoop out the seeds. Place face-down on a baking pan, lightly oiled with the olive oil. Bake 25-30 minutes, until flesh is tender.
3. While squash is baking, bring the carrots, turnips, and apples to a boil in a saucepan over high heat. Cook about 20 minutes, until tender. Drain the vegetables and return them to the pot.
4. Remove the squash from the oven and scoop out the flesh, using a spoon. Add the squash to the other vegetables. Do not turn off the oven.

5. Add the coconut oil, cinnamon, and salt to the pot. Mash using a potato masher or electric mixer.
6. Scoop the vegetable mixture into the 4 squash shells.
7. Return the squash to the baking dish and bake uncovered until heated through, about 15-20 minutes.

Purple Plum Cabbage

Prep Time: 10 minutes

Cook Time: 10 minutes

Servings: 4

INGREDIENTS

1 head purple cabbage, halved, cored, and sliced into thin ribbons

3 Tablespoons olive oil

3 Tablespoons umeboshi plum vinegar (can substitute cider vinegar)

INSTRUCTIONS

1. Bring a large pot of water to a boil over high heat. Add the cabbage and boil for 3-5 minutes.
2. Drain the cabbage and rinse with cold water.
3. Add the cabbage to a large bowl and toss with the vinegar and oil (this is easiest with your hands).

Coconut Cauliflower

Prep Time: 10 minutes

Cook Time: 10 minutes

Servings: 4

INGREDIENTS

1 head cauliflower, chopped

½ cup coconut milk

1 Tablespoon coconut oil

½ teaspoon turmeric

¼ teaspoon ground cinnamon

½ teaspoon sea salt

INSTRUCTIONS

1. Bring a large pot of water to a boil over high heat. Add the cauliflower and boil for 5-7 minutes, until soft.
2. Drain the cauliflower and return it to the pot.
3. Add the coconut milk, oil, and spices, and mash with a potato masher.

Roasted Brussels Sprouts

Prep Time: 15 minutes

Cook Time: 30 minutes

Servings: 4

INGREDIENTS

2 pounds Brussels sprouts

3 Tablespoons olive oil

4 slices bacon, chopped

1 teaspoon sea salt

INSTRUCTIONS

1. Preheat oven to 400 °F.
2. Trim the ends off of the Brussels sprouts and cut into quarters.
3. Place in a roasting pan with the bacon, oil, and salt, and toss until mixed.
4. Roast for 20 minutes. Continue roasting, checking frequently, until just browned. It can take up to 30 minutes to reach desired level of doneness.

Braised Sweet Potatoes and Kale

Prep Time: minutes

Cook Time: minutes

Servings: 4

INGREDIENTS

4 sweet potatoes, peeled and chopped

1 Tablespoon coconut oil

1 yellow onion, chopped

1 large bunch kale, chopped

½ cup chicken broth

1 orange

1 Tablespoon apple cider vinegar

½ teaspoon sea salt

INSTRUCTIONS

1. Bring potatoes to a boil in a large saucepan over high heat. Lower to a simmer and cook until potatoes are tender, about 15 minutes.

2. Heat the oil in a large, deep-sided sauté pan. Add the onion and sauté until translucent, about 5 minutes.

3. Add the kale to the pan, and stir.

4. Add the sweet potatoes. Pour the broth over the vegetables, cover, and cook until kale is cooked through, about 5 minutes.

5. Juice the orange into a bowl. Add the vinegar and the salt and whisk together. Pour over the vegetable mixture.

Sautéed Snap Peas and Mushrooms

Prep Time: 10 minutes

Cook Time: 10 minutes

Servings: 4

INGREDIENTS

1 pound snap peas

10-12 ounces mushrooms, halved

1 shallot, thinly sliced

2 Tablespoons olive oil

Sea salt to taste

INSTRUCTIONS

1. Remove the stem and the "string" from each pea pod.
2. Sauté the shallot in the olive oil in a skillet over high heat for 2-3 minutes.
3. Add the mushrooms and sauté, stirring, for about 4-5 minutes.
4. Add the snap peas and sauté 2-3 more minutes, until the peas are crisp –tender. Add salt to taste.

Summer Squash Medley

Prep Time: minutes

Cook Time: minutes

Servings: 4

INGREDIENTS

1 large yellow summer squash

1 large zucchini

2 Tablespoons olive oil

¼ cup fresh parsley leaves, chopped

Sea salt to taste

INSTRUCTIONS

1. Slice the squash into half-rounds.
2. Sauté the oil in a large skillet and add the squash and parsley. Cook for 10-12 minutes, stirring frequently. Add salt to taste.

Chapter 3

Snacks

Anti-Inflammatory Mango Smoothie

Prep Time: 5 minutes

Cook Time: N/A

Servings: 1

INGREDIENTS

1 banana, fresh or frozen

1 mango, peeled and chopped

1 cup coconut water

1 Tablespoon coconut oil

1 teaspoon turmeric

½ teaspoon cinnamon

½ teaspoon ground ginger

INSTRUCTIONS

1. Add all ingredients to the blender and blend until smooth.

Green Coconut Smoothie

Prep Time: 5 minutes

Cook Time: N/A

Servings: 1

INGREDIENTS

1 avocado, peeled and chopped

1 green apple, chopped

1 Tablespoon coconut oil

½ cup coconut milk or coconut water

1 cup fresh spinach

½ teaspoon ground ginger

1 lime, juiced

INSTRUCTIONS

1. Add all ingredients to the blender and blend until smooth.

Minty Melon Smoothie

Prep Time: 5 minutes

Cook Time: N/A

Servings: 1

INGREDIENTS

1 cantaloupe half, peeled and chopped

1 peach, pitted and chopped

½ cup coconut milk or coconut water

1 Tablespoon coconut oil

10 leaves fresh mint

INSTRUCTIONS

1. Add all ingredients to the blender and blend until smooth.

Warming Turmeric Tea

Prep Time: 5 minutes

Cook Time: 5

Servings: 1

INGREDIENTS

1 cup coconut milk

1 teaspoon turmeric

1 teaspoon ground cinnamon

1 inch fresh ginger, peeled (or ½ teaspoon ground ginger)

INSTRUCTIONS

1. Add all ingredients to a small sauce pan and bring to a simmer over low heat, stirring frequently. Do not bring to a boil.

2. Pour the tea through a mesh strainer to remove the ginger and serve.

Mojito Mocktails

Prep Time: 5 minutes

Cook Time: N/A

Servings: 8

INGREDIENTS

1 large cucumber, sliced

1 lime, thinly sliced

½ cup fresh mint leaves

64 ounces filtered water or unflavored soda water

ice

INSTRUCTIONS

1. Add lime and mint to a large pitcher.
2. Add ice and stir to slightly crush the mint and lime.
3. Add the cucumber slices and water.
4. Chill until ready to serve

www.ingramcontent.com/pod-product-compliance
Lightning Source LLC
Chambersburg PA
CBHW051224170526
45166CB00005B/2030